I0844983

10 Pounds In 14 Days

A Step by Step No Fluff Guide To Losing Weight Fast!

by Kurt Tasche

All Rights Reserved. No part of this publication may be reproduced in any form or by any means, including scanning, photocopying, or otherwise without prior written permission of the copyright holder. Copyright © 2020

Table of Contents

10 Pounds In 14 Days

by Kurt Tasche

Dedication

This book is dedicated to my husband Micheal, who has supported me through all of life's ups and downs.

Disclaimer

The information contained in this book is based on the author's personal experience and is not meant to substitute any professional or medical advice.

The reader assumes all responsibility and shall not hold the author or publisher responsible for any repercussions or consequences due to the use or misuse of this information.

It is highly suggested that the reader seek the advice of a medical professional before beginning any diet or exercise program.

Introduction

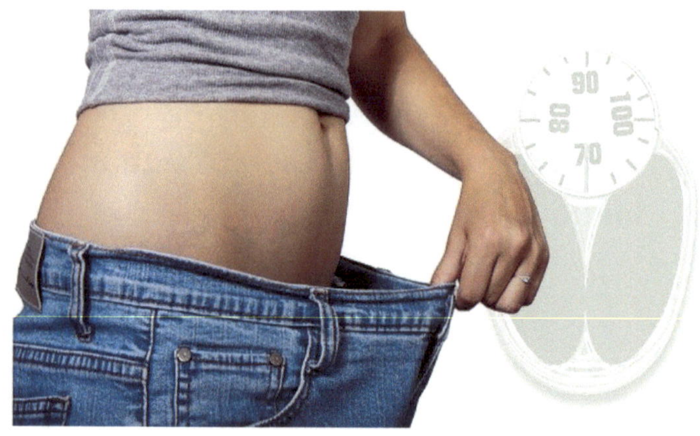

If you ask anyone what their biggest goals are
in life, almost every single one of them will
give you some sort of weight loss goal as their
top (or at least in the top 5) of their most
desired goals. And understandably so.

Weight loss is the number one most searched
topic online, the most profitable industry in the
world, and it is the number one New Year's
resolution every single year.

But why is that?

Why is weight loss the number one searched
topic in the world, the number one industry in

the world, and the number one New Year's resolution every single new year?

Let's be honest.

If people were actually losing weight, then these same people wouldn't keep making these resolutions over and over again. Year after year.

And, the weight loss industry would not be generating over $100 billion annually.

The fact is that, weight loss has become such a convoluted and confusing topic, that people tend to jump from one weight loss program to another, one diet to another, one course to another, one gym to another, one trainer to another, etc, etc.

Until finally, they just give up.

Then, after awhile, they'll find something else, try it, and then either quit or not get the results they want.

Another thing is that, for most people, most weight loss programs are just too hard. They require alot more effort than people really want to put in. Because of society's overall "instant gratification" mindset, we assume that everything we do is going to be super easy and give us instant results. Or, that it will be completely automated, where we won't have to put forth any effort.

But, that's not the case with weight loss. However, it's not as complicated as most people make it out to be.

Weight Loss Is Math

Losing weight is a simple mathematical process. All you have to do is burn more calories than you're taking in, and you'll lose weight. Simple.

The type of exercises you're doing or the type of food you're eating, has little to do with this.

It's simply math.

Now obviously, exercising and eating healthy are going to help and will optimize your weight loss greatly.

If you can understand this simple mathematical equation, which is:

Eat Less and Move More...

You will lose weight.

However, there's always a way we can help this along.

10.2 lbs In Just 14 Days

When I decided to start my own weight loss journey, I wasn't really obese. But I was a bit overweight.

I had, up until high school, weighed as high as 155 lbs. Which really wasn't that bad.

Then in 2011-2012, I was diagnosed with cancer (non-Hodgkin's Lymphoma) and as a side effect of chemotherapy, I lost a lot of weight.

The idea was, after I felt better, to start eating more to gain weight back. But instead of eating healthy, I was eating a bunch of junk. I was eating carbs, deep fried foods, pastries, chips. Anything I could get my hands on, I was eating.

I wasn't eating like I should.

So what happened then was, I went from being underweight at about 110 lbs, and ate myself to around 190 lbs.

After a few years of walking 3 miles a day, eating better, cutting down on the carbs, etc. I still wasn't getting the results I wanted. I ended up getting down to 167 lbs, but I was stuck there. I couldn't get passed that. Nothing else was working.

Then finally, a friend of mine sent me an email about something he was doing that helped him lose alot of weight. I think he said he lost 60 lbs within a month or two.

So I decided to give it a shot.

In this book, I'm going to explain to you exactly what it is that I did. I'll explain to you exactly how I lost 10.2 lbs in 14 days.

Yes, the title of this book is "10 lbs in 14 Days". However, the exact amount of weight I lost was 10.2 lbs.

So, I went from 167 lbs to 156.8 lbs in 14 days.

Then, a few weeks after that, I dropped myself down to 145 lbs.

Now, I know what you're thinking:

"Sure Kurt. It worked for you. But will it work for me?"

My answer to that is, absolutely yes!

But ONLY if you follow the steps in this guide EXACTLY as I've laid them out for you.

You have to follow the plan in front of you.

A blueprint is not designed to be altered, especially while you are following it.

For example, if you're building a house, and you decide to alter the blueprint during construction (even the smallest thing) the house is not going to turn out the same way. In fact, it might not even stand.

The same goes for this program. You must follow the blueprint exactly in order to get the results you want.

Now, will you get the exact same results as me? I don't know. Everyone's body is different. Everyone's dedication and commitment is different. So, it's all going to depend upon you.

But I have confidence that, if you follow the plan and stay consistent, you will get results. You will lose weight.

With that, let's move on to Chapter One.

Chapter 1: Mindset

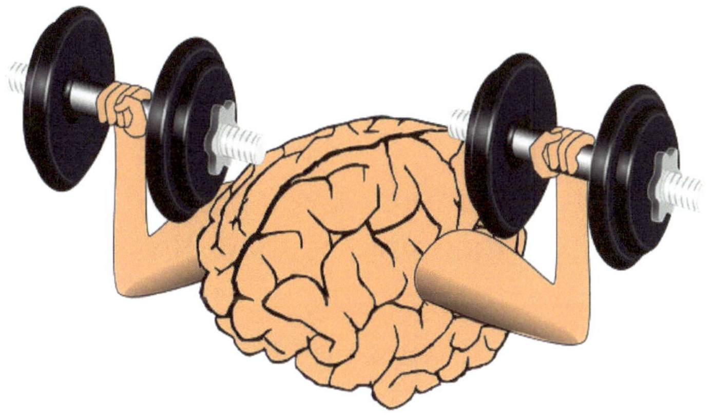

Now, before we get into the meat of this program, I want to stress to you the importance of mindset. Because, if you don't have your mind right, you're not going to get the results you want.

Everything starts with belief. If you don't believe you can lose weight, then you won't take the actions necessary in order to do so. However, if you do believe, then there's no stopping you.

Now to be more clear and detailed, there's a part of the brain called the *Reticular Activating System* (RAS). And what this does is determine what you pay attention to in the world. And that is based on your beliefs.

So for example, if you believe you cannot lose weight, then your RAS will focus on and pick up everything in the world that's going to prove to you that what you believe is true. In this case, that you *cannot* lose weight.

However, if you believe strongly that you can lose weight, then your Reticular Activating System will pick up and focus on all the things around you, that are going to prove to you that *you can do it.*

You see, your mind, through the RAS, is going to prove to you, that whatever you believe is true. And this goes for anything in your life. But in our case with weight loss, if you believe you can do it, then you absolutely will do it.

The BAR Trifecta

I came up with a concept called "The BAR Trifecta", which I'll be writing a separate book on in the very near future.

BAR stands for:
1. Beliefs
2. Actions
3. Results

And based upon the Reticular Activating System, if you believe something, you'll take the actions necessary to accomplish that thing. For example, weight loss. If you believe you can lose weight, you will take the actions necessary. And of course, the actions, are the plans in this book.

Once you take those actions, you'll get a result. Now, that result is going to reinforce and strengthen your beliefs. Those strengthened beliefs will cause you to take bolder, stronger and more consistent actions. Those stronger actions will produce even better results. Which will strengthen your beliefs even more.

This cycle continues to strengthen itself over and over and over again, and does not stop, as long as you keep going. As long as you don't remove any of the three elements (beliefs, actions or results).

If you stop believing, you'll stop taking action, which won't give you any results.

If you believe, but don't take action, results aren't going to happen.

Writing Down Your Goals

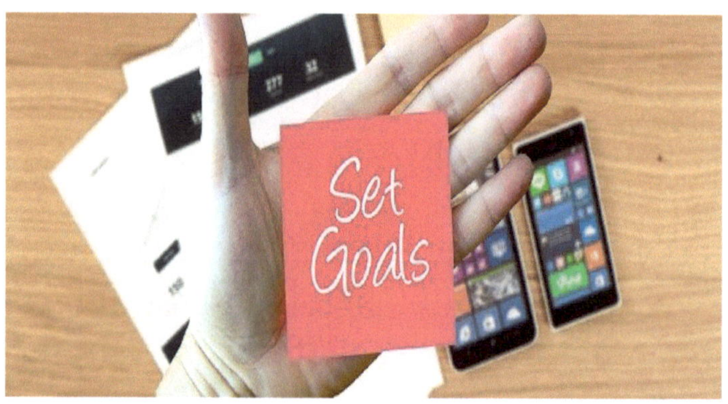

Before we get started, what I want you to do, is get out a sheet of paper and write down your weight loss goal.

But, I don't want you to write it down as what you want to lose. I want you to write it down as what you want to weigh, and write it in the present tense.

For example, if you currently weigh 200 lbs, and you want to lose 50 lbs, I want you to write down on a piece of paper, with emotion:

"I am so happy and grateful that I now weigh 150 lbs and am healthy and happy." Or something to that effect.

Then I want you to think about how long you believe it will take you to lose 50 lbs.

Now, if you've lost 50 lbs in the past, then you have an idea of how long it should take you. For example, lets say it took you 2 months to lose 50 lbs before, then that would be a very realistic time frame for you, based on your past experience.

If you've never lost weight before, then you'll have to adjust this time to suit your own situation. The exact time will be unique to each individual.

So let's say you believe that you can drop 50 lbs in 2 months. And let's say that the date 2 months from now will be July 24, 2020. What I want you to do is, after you've written down your weight loss goal as I mentioned earlier ("I am so happy and grateful that I now weigh 150 lbs and am healthy and happy.") I want you to write the words: "Today's Date: July 24, 2020" (or whatever your target date is.)

So for example, if your target date is July 24, 2020, then I want you to write it as such:

"I am so happy and grateful that I now weigh 150 lbs and am healthy and happy."
Today's Date: July 24, 2020

Of course, adjust that according to your own weight loss goal and time frame.

If you're still having trouble coming up with a target date, you can use the title of this book as a guide. For example, it took me 14 days to lose 10 lbs. So, mathematically speaking, losing 50 lbs may have take me 70 days (or about 3 months, 10 days).

The idea is not to try and be "correct" by guessing when you'll reach your weight loss goal, but to give you a deadline to provide that extra push and motivation to finish what you started. Too many goals go unfulfilled because people just aren't motivated enough to see them through to the end.

Now you may be wondering why we are writing our goals in this format. It's because we want to write our goals in the present tense. We want you to get your mindset, body, etc. in the feeling and state of already having achieved your goal. Because when you get yourself into the feeling of already achieving your goal, it's going to allow you to pick up, focus on and attract everything in the world that will help you make accomplishing that goal and make it a reality.

Basically, it will super-charge your Reticular Activating System to deliberately focus on and find those things necessary to achieve your weight loss goal.

Now this is just a small part of our whole weight loss program. The rest of this program is very simple and direct, with no fluff. I want you to get the best results as quickly as possible.

This program is not confusing like other weight loss plans you may have tried in the past.

You're not going to be counting calories.
You're not going to be doing hundreds of
jumping jacks or push-ups, or running 5 miles
a day, or anything like that.

You're simply going to be following a plan,
sticking with it, and getting results.

With that said, let's get into the program!

Chapter 2: Drink This First!

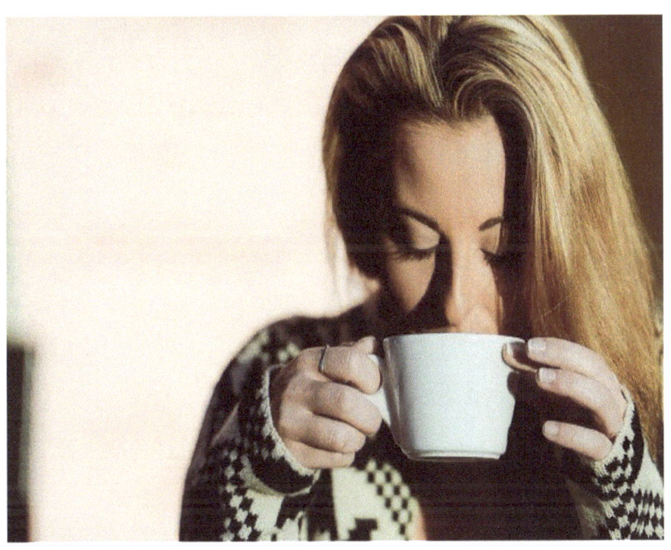

Many weight loss programs include some sort of beverage. Either juices, smoothies, shakes, potions or other drinks, that are designed to help you lose weight.

And although many of these are great products, and many give great results, the fact of the matter is the reason why most people can't lose weight with these programs is because these products are not something most people drink on a regular basis.

They are something you have to add to your diet, train yourself to actually drink, and sometimes even train yourself (and trick yourself) into liking them. Many of these products are just absolutely awful tasting. And most people don't stick with these programs because of this.

But, what if it didn't have to be this way?

What if you could lose weight by drinking something every day, that you already drink? Something that's part of your regular routine already.

You wouldn't have to change anything. You'd simply have to keep doing what you're already doing.

Now, isn't that a novel concept?

This one thing is the reason why I was able to lose 10 lbs (or more precisely, 10.2 lbs) in just 14 days.

Something that I already do on a regular basis, and that virtually every single person (or atleast, most people) already do on a daily basis anyway.

Now, what is that one thing?

That one thing is...

Coffee

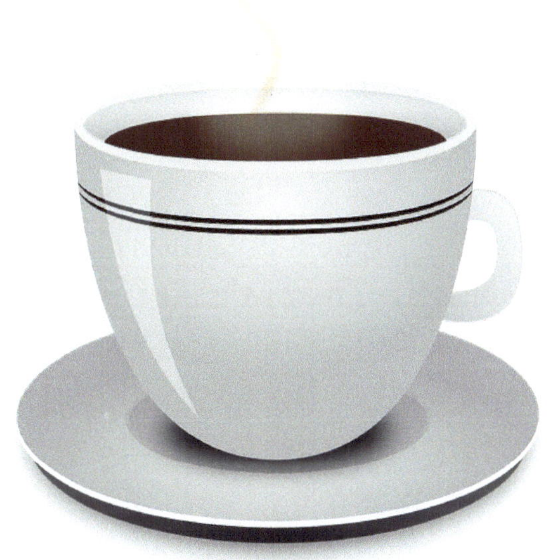

But not just any coffee.

This is a special coffee that is designed to help you lose weight!

Now, I know what you're thinking. You've seen plenty of weight loss coffees in the past. They all are super gross tasting, they get you overly amped up, most of them give you headaches, you feel like your heart's gonna pound out of your chest, and they're just absolutely awful.

And no one in their right mind would keep drinking them. Which is why hardly anyone gets results.

But that's not the case here.

First of all, this coffee is actually *REAL COFFEE*. Most weight loss coffees aren't coffee at all. They're a combination of herbs, roots and other things that are meant to mimic coffee. But they are just not coffee.

This is actual coffee, with special ingredients, that block the hunger signals in your brain, as well as the craving signals that cause you to crave junk foods.

You see, the reason why most people are having trouble losing weight, is because they have an addiction to carbohydrates. More specifically, incomplete carbs (junk foods such as chips, cookies, pastries, etc), things that are high in sugar and white flour. Foods that your body will store as fat, if it doesn't use those carbs right away. And, if you're not a world-class athlete, you're storing most or all of those carbs as fat.

Another challenge people have when trying to lose weight, is that most people are addicted to eating huge portions of food. And, it doesn't matter if those large portions are made up of healthy foods. When you eat too much, you'll keep gaining weight.

What this coffee does, is it first blocks the hunger signals in your brain that causes you to want to eat. It actually blocks that signal that your brain sends to your stomach, that tells it you are hungry. It also blocks those cravings, those signals, that make you crave carbs and junk food.

By doing this, you'll take in less of these bad foods, and less food in general, and you'll lose weight. Your body will actually use the fat is has stored for energy.

Now to learn more, and to get yourself some of this special coffee, simply visit the website below:

http://www.slimcoffee.xyz

With that being said, order yourself some of the coffee, and we'll continue with the next chapter.

Chapter 3: Here's How It Works

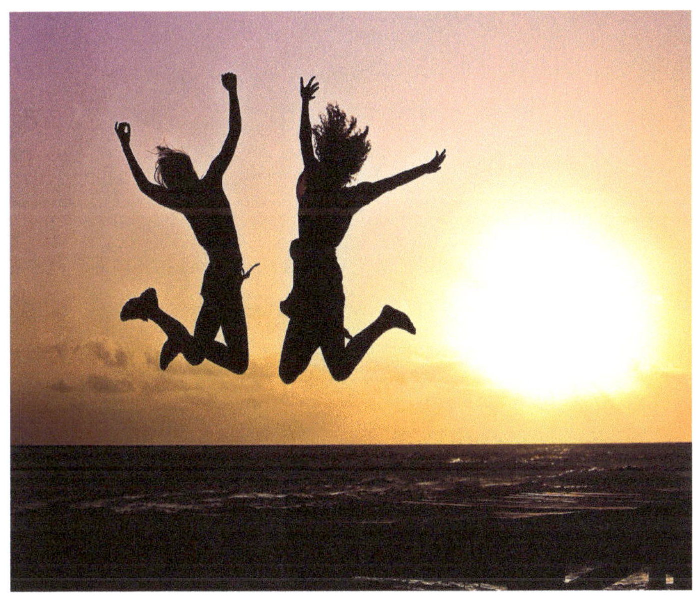

Now, if you've already gotten yourself some of the special coffee that I talked about in Chapter 2, you're probably wonder, how do you use it to get the best results?

Well, it's a very simple process the we're gonna go over right now. Like I said earlier, I don't want to have this book filled with any fluff, because I want you to get the best results as quickly as possible.

So, let's get to it!

First thing in the morning, when you wake up, you're going to have one cup of the coffee, on an empty stomach. Then you're gonna wait atleast 90 minutes after you've finished your coffee, before you decide to eat anything.

This gives time for the ingredients in the coffee to take effect, so they'll do what they are meant to do. And what they're going to do is:

1. Block the hunger signals that the brain sends to your stomach.
2. Block the craving signals that cause you to want carbs and junk foods.
3. Keep you more focused.
4. Metabolize the fat you have stored better, so your body can use that fat as energy more efficiently.

Now after 90 minutes is up, if you decide to eat anything, that's fine. However, I do know people (including myself) who are using the coffee, who don't eat breakfast at all. All they do is have their coffee in the morning with no breakfast, a small lunch, and then a medium to small dinner.

So, let's do a quick recap:

1. Wake up and have one cup of the coffee first thing, on an empty stomach. (You're not gonna have your coffee with a stack of pancakes! That's going to defeat the purpose.)
2. Wait at least 90 minutes after you've finished the coffee before you decide to eat anything. If you don't feel hungry, then don't force yourself to eat. This is completely up to you.

The reason why some people don't need to eat any breakfast after having the coffee, is because the energy they need is coming from the fat that is already stored on their body. And using stored fat as energy is one of the main keys of weight loss.

So now that you know what to do, and how to use the coffee to lose weight, you're probably wondering, if the coffee is blocking hunger and craving signals, what exactly should I be eating?

Well, you may be surprised to learn that , there's no real rule to this.

But, will get into the details in the next chapter.

Chapter 4: What Can I Eat?

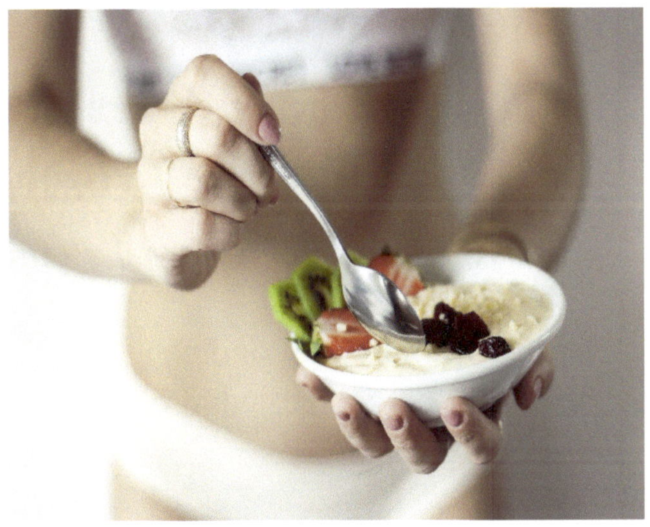

Now, if you've been using the coffee as I mentioned in the last chapter, you should soon be feeling the effects that are going to assist you in losing weight. Those effects being:

1. The hunger signals that your brain sends to your stomach are blocked. Therefore, you won't be as hungry as you might normally be.

2. The craving signals are blocked.
   Therefore, you won't be craving things
   like carbs and junk food.
3. The fat in your body will be metabolized
   better. That way, you burn fat more
   easily,
4. You'll begin to feel more focused.
5. You'll have more energy.

And, you'll just feel better all around.

Now you may be wondering, now that you're drinking the coffee, what can you eat and still lose weight?

What do you need to avoid? What foods can you have?

Well, you may be surprised to learn that, there really is no rule to what you can eat.

You see, drinking the coffee is going to cause you to eat less anyway. So no matter what you eat, you're going to eat less. This way, you'll lose weight. Like I said before, weight loss is simple mathematics. You burn more calories than you take in, and you lose weight.

With the coffee being drank first thing in the morning, on an empty stomach, you will not be as hungry during the day, you will eat less, you will burn more calories, and you will lose weight.

However, if you want to maximize your results, you can opt to cut out more carbs.

For complete transparency, one of the reasons I lost weight so fast, is that I decided I was going to cut out most, if not all, carbs from my diet.

Now you can still lose weight and still get similar results (or even better results) depending upon how you go about this, if you still eat some carbs. My recommendation however, is to eat as healthy as you can.

Either way you go about this, as long as you stick with drinking the coffee each morning as instructed, you will lose weight.

So, to recap:

1. Drink the coffee first thing in the morning on an empty stomach.

2. Wait atleast 90 minutes after you've finished your coffee before you decide to eat anything.
3. When you do eat, you'll consume smaller meals, because you won't be as hungry.

Again, there really are no rules as to what you can eat with this program. If you decide to cut out some things, by all means do so. I would say, if you are going to cut out some foods, cut out alot of the empty calorie (junk) foods, bad or "incomplete" carbs, white flour-based foods, etc. Do this and you'll get results even faster.

So now that you've learned that there's really no rule to what you can eat with this program, the next step is learning how to burn the most calories possible each day. What type of exercises should you be doing to lose weight the fastest?

Well, we're going to answer that question in the next chapter.

Chapter 5: Exercise

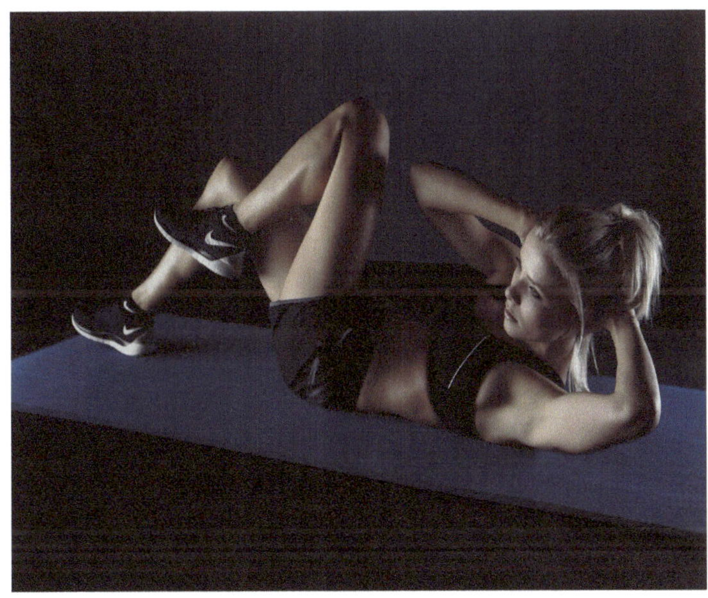

Weight loss is nothing but simple math. You just burn more calories than you take in, and you will lose weight.

That being said, you may be wondering, what type of exercises you need to do with this program, to get the most benefit.   Well, you'll be surprised to know that, there really is no rule. But, I'm going to give you some suggestions and tips to help you get the maximum benefit.

First of all, you're going to be burning calories anyway. Since you're taking in less calories because of the coffee, you're going to lose weight regardless of exercise.

But lets say you work a job that requires alot of moving around. By doing your every day routine, you'll be burning even more calories. And because the coffee helps your body metabolize fat better, you'll be losing more weight than if you didn't drink the coffee.

No matter what type of exercise or movement you do, I suggest setting a goal of taking at least 10,000 steps per day.

If you need help tracking your steps, there are plenty of free and paid devices and services you can use such as Google Fit, FitBit, Samsung Health and others.

Even without taking 10,000 steps a day, you will still lose weight, because you are taking in less calories than you normally would.

Also, if you have a favorite sport or other physical activity that you like to do, that's definitely going to increase your calorie burning by leaps and bounds. Whether you're into tennis, racket ball, running, martial arts, rock climbing or whatever it is, physical activity will help you lose weight even faster.

So again, there's no hard and fast rule on what exercise(s) you need to do. You don't need to do 100 jumping jacks or an hour of intense aerobics each day. All you need to do, is what you normally do throughout the day.

Whether you're working, playing your favorite sport, or whatever it is, set a goal of 10,000 steps a day, and that's going to give you the most benefit and optimum results.

But, that being said, no one person is an island. It's much easier to get results when you have someone to work with. A partner.

In the next chapter, we're going to talk about getting yourself an accountability partner. Someone who has similar goals as you, who will work with you, so you can both help keep each other on track.

We'll get into all that in the next chapter.

Chapter 6: Partner Up!

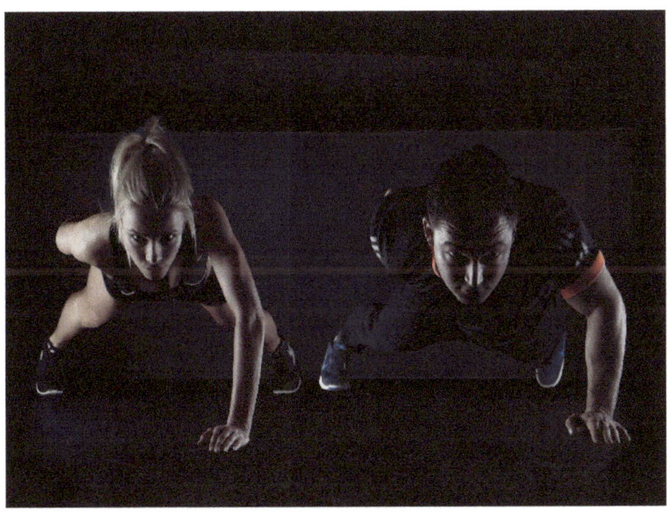

Now weight loss can be a huge challenge, especially when you're going about it by yourself. You have to keep your self motivated, hold yourself accountable, and keep yourself on track to get the results you want.

One of the best ways to get results even faster, with anything in life, is to have an accountability partner. Somebody who has similar goals as you, who also wants to lose weight, and is willing to work this program with you. That way, you can both motivate and hold each other accountable to get the results you both want.

SPECIAL BONUS: We have created a special Facebook Group for those who want to maximize their results with this program. This group is designed to make it easier for you to find an accountability partner (or partners) and includes many other benefits. You can request to join the group here:

https://www.facebook.com/groups/10pounds in14days/

The first thing you need to do, in order to make this work, is to be sure that both of you are willing to get the special coffee. Again, you can get the coffee here: http://slimcoffee.xyz

Then, every morning, either call, text each other, or talk face to face, to make sure you are both drinking the coffee as instructed. How you communicate each morning will depend on whether you both live in the same or separate households.

Next, keep track of the amount of exercise and movement you're both doing throughout the day. Keep yourself and your partner motivated to take atleast 10,000 steps per day.

Also, if you and your partner decide to cut out certain foods, make sure that you and your partner are both making sure that you are both following your own chosen eating plan. Because of different tastes and situations, you and your partner may not cut out the same foods. Be sure you both have a clear understanding of the other's plan so you can help each other stay on point.

This way you can both work the program, drink the coffee, and achieve the results you each want, in less time than it would take if you did it all on your own.

Remember, the point of having an accountability partner is to hold you accountable, But it's also to help motivate and encourage you to keep going.

So talk to your friends, family and anyone else who wants to lose weight and see if you can get them to become accountability partners with you. In fact, you can have a group of accountability partners, all helping each other.

In Chapter 7 we'll do a recap of the entire program. See you then!

Chapter 7: Recap

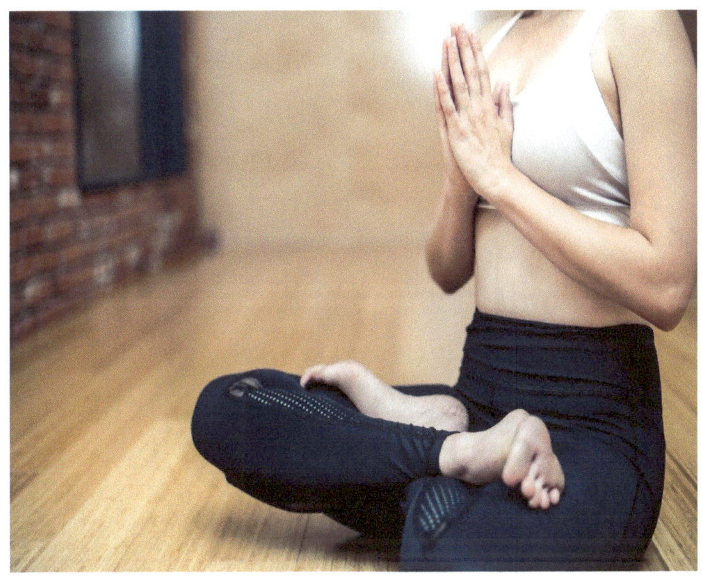

Now that you've gone through the last 6 chapters, it's time to do a quick recap, to make sure you understand how to work this program to get the maximum benefit.

First - Keep yourself in a positive state of mind. Keep your mindset right. You need to make sure that you're in the right frame of mind in order for this program to work for you. You must believe and know, for certain, that it's going to work.

If you doubt yourself, you'll begin filling your head with negative self-talk, and you won't follow through. I suggest, everyday, listening to motivational speakers like Les Brown, Tony Robbins, Bob Proctor, Brian Tracy, and others, who will help keep you in a positive state-of-mind to keep you on the right track.

Second - Always be sure you are drinking your coffee, one or two cups in the morning on an empty stomach, and then waiting at least 90 minutes before you decide to have any food. Again, you can get your coffee at:
http://slimcoffee.xyz

Third - If you opt to cut out any foods, look at cutting out white flour foods, empty carbs and other foods that are known to be the enemies of fat loss. Remember, there is no actual need to cut out any foods, but you will optimize your results by removing as much junk from your diet as possible.

Fourth - As far as exercising goes, there is no set rule as to what you must do. You will lose weight regardless, because you are taking in less calories (all thanks to the coffee). However, taking at least 10,000 steps per day, as recommended in Chapter 5, will super-charge your calorie-burning power, so you lose weight even faster.

How you take those 10,000 steps is completely up to you. Whether you do it by walking, working your job, playing your favorite sport, etc, does not matter. Just set that goal, and you will succeed.

<u>Fifth</u> - Find yourself an accountability partner. Now, you can do the program on your own. That's fine. However, I've found that having a partner helps keep you motivated, holds you accountable, and helps keep you on track to see this through to the end.

Find someone who has similar weight loss goals as you, partner with them, and keep each other focused on your goals. You can find accountability partners and keep yourself motivated by joining our exclusive Facebook Group:
https://www.facebook.com/groups/10pounds in14days

So, now it's time to get to work.

You've set your goals.
You know what you want.
You know what you have to do.

Now, let's just do it!

About The Author

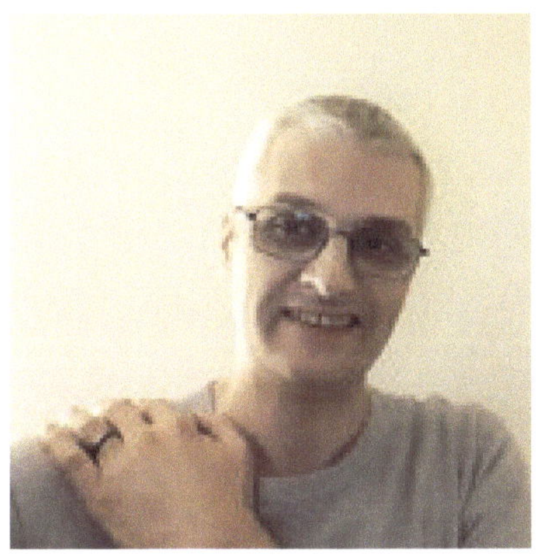

Kurt Tasche was born March 24, 1970 in Hammond, Indiana. He is a cancer survivor, author, speaker, entrepreneur, martial artist and certified personal trainer.

Kurt began his study of Fitness & Nutrition in 1994. From there, he developed a passion for various aspects of health and exercise, including: weight loss, yoga, martial arts, weight training, and more.

Along with fitness and health, Kurt also writes on the topics of personal development (law of attraction, NLP, subconcious reprogramming

and more) as well as entrepreneurship (internet
marketing, home business, and more.)

To see Kurt's full list of published books,
please visit his Author Page at:
http://amazon.com/author/kurttasche

Follow Kurt on Social Media:
http://about.me/kurttasche

Resources

Special Weight Loss Coffee:
http://slimcoffee.xyz

10 Pounds In 14 Days Facebook Group:
https://www.facebook.com/groups/10poundsin14days

More From This Author:
http://amazon.com/author/kurttasche

Follow Kurt: http://about.me/kurttasche

www.ingramcontent.com/pod-product-compliance
Lightning Source LLC
Chambersburg PA
CBHW040238240726
48664CB00001B/182